RESTORING GUT HEALTH FOR WOMEN

A Comprehensive Guide to Digestive Wellness, Probiotics, Balanced Diet, and Stress Management for Women – Unlocking Long-Term Vitality and Preventing Gut Issues

Elsa P. Benson

ABOUT THE AUTHOR

Elsa P. Benson, the creative mind behind the transforming book 'Restoring Gut Health for Women,' is a seasoned specialist in the disciplines of nutrition and women's health. With a wealth of knowledge gathered through years of focused study and hands-on experience, Elsa has become a recognized expert in leading women toward maximum well-being through the lens of gut health.

Elsa offers advanced degrees in Nutrition and Integrative Health, combining scientific rigor with a holistic approach to help women in recovering their vitality. Her enthusiasm for deciphering the subtleties of the gut-body link and its significant influence on hormonal balance inspired her to write this thorough guide geared exclusively for women.

Having worked with many cultures and people on their health journeys, Elsa knows the particular needs and problems women experience across different life phases. the knowledge goes beyond theory, as she adds practical ideas and feasible techniques to the pages of the book.

With 'Restoring Gut Health for Women,' Elsa P. Benson takes readers into a world where the confluence of diet, hormones, and gut health provides a path for lifelong vitality. Elsa's work displays not just her competence but also her real desire to enable women to take care of their health.

As a sought-after speaker, educator, and champion for women's well-being, Elsa P. Benson continues to inspire countless others to go on their transforming journeys. Her book serves as a tribute to her devotion to spreading information that can improve lives.

Follow Elsa on this illuminating journey into the world of gut health and learn how her counsel may pave the path for a healthier, more vibrant you. With Elsa P. Benson as your trusted companion, go on a road of rehabilitation, empowerment, and sustained well-being.

CONTENTS

INTRODUCTION

In a society filled with fast-paced lives, changing diets, and growing stress, the relevance of gut health has emerged as a beacon of well-being. This is a book devoted to a wonderful journey, one that goes deep into the complicated realm of gut health and its profound relationship to women's overall health.

The human gut, that small but incredibly intricate ecosystem hidden inside us, plays a critical role in our health and vitality. For women, knowing and cultivating this often-overlooked part of their well-being is not simply an issue of physical health but a gateway to empowerment and a greater quality of life.

In the pages that follow, we will investigate the complex interaction between the stomach and the female body, exposing the secrets of how gut health influences everything from hormone balance to immune function. We will learn to identify common gut health disorders that disproportionately impact women, and we'll engage on a road of healing and restoration.

From food choices to stress management, exercise to preventative measures, this book is your entire guide to restoring and maintaining excellent gut health. We'll uncover the tasty and nutritious meals that may relax and revitalize your gut, and we'll examine the ways to guarantee that your gut stays a source of strength, resilience, and well-being throughout your life's various phases.

The power to heal, the ability to flourish, and the power to restore control over your health starts inside your gut. Welcome to a world where your gut is not just a passive spectator but an active player in your life's symphony. Let's go on this adventure together, as we unearth the keys of restoring gut health for women.

UNDERSTANDING THE IMPORTANCE OF GUT HEALTH

Recognizing the significance of gut health is vital for sustaining overall well-being. The gut, sometimes referred to as the "second brain," is a complex and essential system that extends beyond merely digesting. It holds billions of bacteria that make up the gut microbiome, which plays a crucial role in different physiological activities.

A healthy gut not only enables effective digestion and absorption of nutrients but also regulates numerous areas of health, including immune function, hormone balance, and even mental well-being. Studies have emphasized the influence of the gut microbiome on the regulation of the immune system, indicating its significance in avoiding autoimmune disorders and allergies.

Furthermore, the gut-brain axis underlines the delicate link between gut health and mental health. Research has demonstrated how abnormalities in the gut microbiota might lead to mood disorders, such as anxiety and depression. Understanding and supporting gut health is therefore vital for preserving not only physical health but also emotional and mental stability.

Moreover, for women particularly, the relevance of gut health extends to hormonal balance and reproductive health. The gut microbiota regulates the metabolism of estrogen and other hormones, underlining its significance in controlling menstrual cycles, fertility, and menopausal transitions.

In short, grasping the significance of gut health extends beyond the scope of digestion; it covers a comprehensive awareness of the body's deep interconnections. By emphasizing gut health, women may pave the path for a stronger immune system, hormonal balance, enhanced mental health, and overall vitality.

WHY GUT HEALTH MATTERS FOR WOMEN

Gut health bears special relevance for women owing to its deep effect on different facets of their well-being. For women, the gut microbiome's equilibrium plays a vital role in maintaining hormonal balance, supporting reproductive health, and enhancing general immunity.

Firstly, the gut microbiome's influence on hormonal homeostasis is critical. It assists in the metabolism of estrogen, progesterone, and other hormones, directly regulating monthly regularity, fertility, and menopausal transitions. Imbalances inside the stomach might disturb these processes, perhaps leading to irregular menstrual cycles, reproductive issues, or worsened menopausal symptoms.

Secondly, the gut's function in maintaining reproductive health cannot be neglected. An appropriate gut environment leads to the absorption of key nutrients required for fetal growth throughout pregnancy. Additionally, a healthy gut flora may minimize the risk of problems such as gestational diabetes and preeclampsia, supporting a better pregnancy journey.

Furthermore, given the natural relationship between the stomach and the immune system, maintaining gut health becomes vital for enhancing women's overall immunity. A healthy gut microbiota helps avoid infections, boosts the body's fight against pathogens, and decreases the risk of autoimmune disorders that affect women more commonly than males.

In summary, emphasizing gut health for women is vital for maintaining hormonal stability, supporting reproductive wellness, and enhancing the body's natural defensive systems. By nourishing and repairing their gut health, women may pave the path to a happier, more resilient, and balanced existence.

CHAPTER 1

THE GUT-BODY CONNECTION

The gut-body link is a remarkable and complicated association between the gastrointestinal system and numerous parts of the human body. This link extends much beyond the gut's fundamental function in digesting; it involves a complex web of connections that impact general health and well-being.

- **Nutrient Absorption**
- **Immune System**
- **Hormonal Balance**: The gut microbiota regulates the metabolism

and regulation of hormones, including sex hormones like estrogen and progesterone. Imbalances in the stomach may alter hormonal homeostasis, possibly leading to a variety of health concerns, especially in women.

- **Neurological Health**: The gut is sometimes referred to as the "second brain" because of the gut-brain axis, a bidirectional communication pathway between the stomach and the brain. It has a substantial influence on mental health and mood control. Disturbances in the stomach may lead to illnesses like anxiety, sadness, and even neurological abnormalities.

- **Inflammation and Chronic Disease**: Chronic inflammation in the stomach may promote systemic inflammation throughout the body, which is a prevalent component in many chronic illnesses, including cardiovascular disease, diabetes, and autoimmune problems. Maintaining gut health may help minimize the risk of these illnesses.

- **Metabolism and Weight Management**

HOW THE GUT AFFECTS OVERALL HEALTH

The gut has a considerable effect on general health, playing a key part in several biological activities beyond merely digesting. Its influence extends to various systems throughout the body, altering everything from immunological function to mental well-being. Understanding how the stomach influences overall health is crucial to maintaining a healthy and flourishing lifestyle.

Immune System Regulation: A large percentage of the immune system is found in the gut. The gut microbiota interacts with the immune cells, helping to control immune responses and defend against dangerous infections. A well-balanced gut environment is vital for maintaining a healthy and functional immune system, avoiding infections, and minimizing the risk of autoimmune illnesses.

Nutrient Absorption and Energy Production: The gut is important for breaking down food and absorbing nutrients, such as vitamins, minerals, and vital fatty acids. Proper nutrient absorption is critical for giving the body the energy and resources it needs to carry out numerous physiological activities, boosting overall vitality and well-being.

Mental and Emotional Health: The gut-brain axis promotes bidirectional communication between the gut and the brain. This relationship regulates mood control, stress reactions, and possibly cognitive performance. A healthy gut environment may lead to increased mental well-being, whereas abnormalities in the gut microbiota have been related to illnesses such as anxiety, depression, and neurodegenerative disorders.

Inflammation and Disease Prevention: A well-balanced gut helps maintain a healthy inflammatory response inside the body. Chronic inflammation, sometimes produced by abnormalities in the gut microbiota, is a prevalent underlying component in several chronic illnesses, including cardiovascular problems, diabetes, and certain autoimmune ailments. Prioritizing gut health may help lower the risk of certain inflammatory-related diseases.

Metabolic Health and Weight Management: The gut microbiota regulates metabolism, altering how the body absorbs and stores energy from meals. An imbalance in gut flora may lead to metabolic abnormalities, possibly leading to weight gain, obesity, and associated metabolic illnesses. Cultivating a broad and healthy gut flora via good food choices may promote optimal metabolic functioning.

GENDER-SPECIFIC CONSIDERATIONS

Gender-specific considerations play a significant role in understanding how numerous health issues, particularly gut health, affect people differently depending on their biological sex. Recognizing these disparities is vital for adapting healthcare methods and treatments to suit particular demands and problems experienced by various genders. When it comes to gut health, numerous gender-specific variables are worth noting:

- **Hormonal Influences**

Reproductive Health Impact: Women's gut health may be impacted by numerous reproductive aspects such as menstruation, pregnancy, and menopause. Hormonal changes throughout these phases might impact gut function and microbiome composition, possibly leading to variations in digestion, nutritional absorption, and immunological responses.

Autoimmune illnesses: Certain autoimmune illnesses, such as irritable bowel syndrome (IBS) and autoimmune diseases like systemic lupus erythematosus (SLE), are more frequent in women. Gender-specific changes in immunological responses and hormonal swings may contribute to variances in the incidence, severity, and symptomatology of various illnesses.

Nutritional Requirements: Women's nutritional requirements may vary from men owing to changes in body composition, hormonal swings, and reproductive health demands. These variations may impact food choices, nutrient absorption, and gut microbiota composition, underscoring the need for individualized dietary advice to maintain optimum gut health in both genders.

CHAPTER 2

GUT HEALTH AND HORMONES

The association between gut health and hormones is a dynamic and nuanced interaction that dramatically affects overall well-being. The stomach plays a critical role in hormonal control, regulating numerous hormones necessary for reproductive health, stress response, metabolism, and more. Here's a deeper look at the intricate interaction between intestinal health and hormones:

Estrogen and Gut Health:
- Metabolism in the Gut: The gut microbiota is involved in the

metabolism of estrogen. Bacterial enzymes in the stomach may alter the enterohepatic circulation, influencing estrogen reabsorption or excretion.

- Estrobolome: Specific gut bacteria in the estrobolome contribute to the metabolism of estrogen, regulating its levels in the body.
- Imbalances and Estrogen Levels: Dysbiosis or an imbalance in the gut microbiota may lead to disturbances in estrogen metabolism, possibly leading to diseases like estrogen dominance or insufficiency.

Progesterone and Gut Health:

- Microbial Influence: Gut microorganisms indirectly impact progesterone levels by contributing to overall hormonal balance. An imbalance in the gut flora may lead to abnormalities in sex hormone levels, particularly progesterone.

- Neurotransmitter Production: Some gut bacteria are involved in the generation of neurotransmitters that control the hypothalamus-pituitary-adrenal (HPA) axis, influencing progesterone production.

Cortisol and Gut Health:

- Hypothalamus-Pituitary-Adrenal (HPA) Axis: The gut microbiota regulates the HPA axis, a critical regulator of cortisol production. Dysbiosis may lead to HPA axis dysregulation, influencing cortisol levels and the body's stress response.

- Inflammation and Stress Response: Chronic inflammation in the stomach, frequently linked with dysbiosis, may cause a stress response influencing cortisol levels.

Insulin and Metabolic Hormones:

- Metabolic Health: The gut microbiome regulates metabolic health, affecting insulin sensitivity and the control of metabolic hormones. Disruptions in the stomach may lead to illnesses like insulin resistance.

Gut-Brain Axis and Neurotransmitters:

- Communication Pathways: The gut interacts bidirectionally with the brain via the gut-brain axis. Gut microorganisms create neurotransmitters that regulate mood, stress, and hormone balance.

- Serotonin Production: Significant levels of serotonin, a neurotransmitter with hormonal activities, are generated in the stomach. Gut health impacts serotonin levels, altering mood and general well-being.

Immune System Modulation:

- Endocrine-Immune Crosstalk: The gut microbiota functions as a mediator in the crosstalk between the endocrine and immune systems. Dysregulation in the stomach may lead to systemic inflammation, compromising hormone balance and immunological function.

Managing Hormonal Balance Through Gut Health

Managing hormonal balance via gut health requires adopting practices that promote a flourishing gut microbiota, enhance digestion, and contribute to overall hormonal well-being. Recognizing the complicated relationship between the gut and hormones allows for focused lifestyle changes to enhance hormonal balance. Here's a guide on controlling hormone balance via intestinal health:

Nourish Your Gut with a Balanced Diet:

- Fiber-Rich Foods: Include a range of fiber-rich foods such as fruits, vegetables, and whole grains. Fiber promotes gastrointestinal motility and the development of healthy gut flora.

- Probiotic-Rich Foods: Incorporate probiotic-rich foods like yogurt, kefir, sauerkraut, and kimchi. Probiotics contribute to a varied and healthy gut microbiota.

Prebiotics for Gut Microbial Health:

- Prebiotic-Rich Foods: Consume foods high in prebiotics, such as garlic, onions, leeks, and asparagus. Prebiotics feed beneficial gut flora, providing a healthy gut environment.

Balanced Fats for Hormonal Support:

- Healthy Fats: Include sources of healthy fats, such as avocados, almonds, and olive oil. These lipids serve a role in hormone synthesis and cellular function.

Limit Processed Foods and Sugar:
- Minimize Processed Foods: Reduce the consumption of processed foods, since they may disturb gut health and lead to inflammation.
- Control Sugar Intake: Limit added sugars, since excessive sugar intake might influence insulin sensitivity and hormonal balance.

Hydration for Digestive and Hormonal Support:

- Adequate Water Intake: Stay hydrated to help digestion and general physiological processes. Water is needed for optimum hormonal balance.

Manage Stress for Hormonal Harmony:

- Stress-Reducing Practices: Incorporate stress-reducing exercises such as meditation, yoga, deep breathing, or mindfulness. Chronic stress may disrupt the HPA axis and hormonal homeostasis.

Regular Physical Activity:

- Moderate Exercise: Engage in frequent, moderate-intensity exercise. Physical exercise increases gastrointestinal motility and helps regulate stress, leading to hormonal well-being.

Adequate Sleep for Hormonal Regulation:

- Prioritize Sleep: Ensure ample and quality sleep. Sleep is vital for hormonal balance, including cortisol and growth hormone.

Limit Exposure to Endocrine Disruptors:

- Reduce Toxin Exposure: Minimize exposure to endocrine-disrupting chemicals found in some plastics, insecticides, and home items. These substances may interfere with hormonal equilibrium.

Regular Health Check-ups:

- Monitor Hormone Levels: Consider frequent health check-ups to monitor hormone levels. Work with healthcare specialists to resolve any imbalances or concerns.

Proactive Healthcare and Consultation:

- Healthcare Guidance: Work proactively with healthcare specialists, including endocrinologists and trained dietitians, to establish a specific strategy for controlling hormonal balance via gut health.

CHAPTER 3

COMMON GUT HEALTH ISSUES

FOR WOMEN

Common gut health concerns for women comprise a spectrum of diseases that may impair the digestive system and, in turn, damage general well-being. Recognizing these disorders is critical for early intervention and the adoption of focused techniques to optimize digestive health. Here are some typical gut health concerns that women may encounter:

Irritable Bowel Syndrome (IBS):

- ***Symptoms***: IBS may include stomach discomfort, bloating, gas, and changes in bowel habits (diarrhea or constipation).

- ***Factors***: Stress, dietary triggers, and hormonal changes may contribute to IBS.

Gastroesophageal Reflux Disease (GERD):

- ***Symptoms***: GERD results in acid reflux, heartburn, and regurgitation of stomach contents into the esophagus.

- ***Triggers***: Certain meals, stress, and lifestyle factors might induce GERD symptoms.

Constipation:

- *Symptoms*: Difficulty in passing stools, infrequent bowel motions, and abdominal pain.

- *Causes*: Inadequate fiber intake, dehydration, and a sedentary lifestyle might lead to constipation.

Inflammatory Bowel Disease (IBD):

- *Types*: Includes Crohn's disease and ulcerative colitis, characterized by persistent inflammation of the digestive system.

- *Symptoms*: Abdominal discomfort, diarrhea, exhaustion, and weight loss are frequent symptoms.

Celiac Disease:

- *Autoimmune Condition*: Celiac disease is an autoimmune illness produced by gluten ingestion.

- *Symptoms*: Digestive problems, combined with weariness, joint discomfort, and skin difficulties, may arise.

Small Intestinal Bacterial Overgrowth (SIBO):

- *Imbalance in Gut Bacteria*: SIBO includes an overgrowth of bacteria in the small intestine.

- *Symptoms*: Bloating, stomach discomfort, diarrhea, and malabsorption of nutrients may ensue.

Gallbladder Issues:

- *Gallstones*: Gallstones may cause pain and discomfort, frequently prompted by dietary variables.

- *Symptoms*: Pain in the upper abdomen, nausea, and vomiting.

Hormonal Influences on Gut Health:

- *Menstrual Cycle Impact*: Hormonal variations throughout the menstrual cycle may alter bowel habits, resulting in changes in bowel movements.

- *Endometriosis*: Endometriosis, a disorder where uterine tissue develops outside the uterus, may impact the digestive organs.

Food Sensitivities:

- ***Triggered Reactions***: Some women may develop stomach difficulties owing to particular dietary sensitivities, such as lactose intolerance or sensitivity to certain FODMAPs.

Pelvic Floor Dysfunction:

- ***Impact on Bowel Function***: Issues with the pelvic floor muscles may lead to bowel control issues and constipation.

- ***Common in Women***: Pelvic floor dysfunction is more frequent in women, particularly after delivery.

Hormonal Changes During Pregnancy:

- ***Digestive Impact***: Hormonal changes during pregnancy might lead to constipation, bloating, and heartburn.

Digestive Disorders

Digestive diseases cover a wide range of ailments that affect the gastrointestinal (GI) system, compromising the body's capacity to effectively digest and absorb nutrients. These illnesses may vary from common and moderate to severe and persistent. Here's an outline of numerous digestive disorders:

1. Gastroesophageal Reflux Disease (GERD):

- Description: Chronic acid reflux occurs when stomach acid rushes back into the esophagus, leading to irritation and inflammation.

- Symptoms: Heartburn, regurgitation, chest discomfort, and trouble swallowing.

2. Irritable Bowel Syndrome (IBS):

- Functional condition: IBS is a functional GI condition characterized by stomach discomfort, bloating, and changes in bowel habits without visible structural damage.

- Symptoms: Abdominal discomfort, diarrhea, constipation, or alternating between the two.

3. Inflammatory Bowel Disease (IBD):

- Types: Includes Crohn's disease and ulcerative colitis, both involving persistent inflammation of the digestive system.

- Symptoms: Abdominal discomfort, diarrhea, weight loss, and weariness.

4. Celiac Disease:

- Autoimmune Disorder: A response to gluten, causing damage to the small intestinal lining.

- Symptoms: Digestive difficulties, combined with weariness, joint discomfort, and skin rashes.

5. Gallstones:

- Formation: Solid particles that develop in the gallbladder and may impede the passage of bile.

- Symptoms: Abdominal discomfort, nausea, vomiting, and jaundice.

6. Pancreatitis:

- Inflammation: Inflammation of the pancreas, commonly caused by gallstones or heavy alcohol intake.

- Symptoms: Abdominal discomfort, nausea, vomiting, and digestive difficulties.

7. Diverticulitis:

- Diverticula Inflammation: Inflammation or infection of tiny pouches in the walls of the colon.

- Symptoms: Abdominal discomfort, fever, and changes in bowel patterns.

8. Peptic Ulcers:

- Ulcer Formation: Open sores that form on the inner lining of the stomach, small intestine, or esophagus.

- Symptoms: Abdominal discomfort, bloating, and nausea.

9. Gastroenteritis:

- Infection or Inflammation: Inflammation of the stomach and intestines, commonly owing to viral or bacterial infections.

- Symptoms: Diarrhea, vomiting, stomach pains, and fever.

10. Lactose Intolerance:

- Digestive Enzyme Deficiency: Inability to digest lactose, the sugar present in milk and dairy products.

- Symptoms: Bloating, gas, diarrhea, and stomach pain after ingesting dairy.

11. Small Intestinal Bacterial Overgrowth (SIBO):

- Bacterial Overgrowth: Excessive bacteria in the small intestine, interrupt proper digestion.

- Symptoms: Bloating, stomach discomfort, diarrhea, and loss of nutrients.

12. Eosinophilic Esophagitis (EoE):

- Immune reaction: Chronic inflammation of the esophagus produced by an allergic reaction.

- Symptoms: Difficulty swallowing, chest discomfort, and food impaction.

13. Functional Dyspepsia:

- Chronic Indigestion: Persistent discomfort or pain in the upper abdomen without an evident reason.

- Symptoms: Bloating, early satiety, and stomach pain.

14. Hemorrhoids:

- Swollen Veins: Swollen blood vessels in the rectum or anus.

- Symptoms: Rectal hemorrhage, pain, and discomfort.

15. Colorectal Cancer:

- Malignant Growth: Cancer that originates in the colon or rectum.

- Symptoms: Changes in bowel habits, blood in stool, stomach discomfort, and accidental weight loss.

Women-Specific Gut Problems

Women may encounter particular digestive disorders that are impacted by elements unique to their biology and life phases.

Hormonal shifts, reproductive health, and pregnancy may lead to unique gastrointestinal issues. Here are several women-specific gastrointestinal problems:

1. Hormonal Influences on Digestion:

- Menstrual Cycle Impact: Hormonal changes throughout the menstrual cycle might alter bowel patterns, resulting in changes in bowel motions, bloating, or abdominal pain.

- Endometriosis: This syndrome, where uterine tissue develops outside the uterus, may impact the digestive organs, producing discomfort and gastrointestinal symptoms.

2. Pregnancy-Related Gut Issues:

- Morning Sickness: Nausea and vomiting, typically encountered during early pregnancy, might compromise digestive comfort.

- Constipation: Hormonal changes and strain on the digestive system may cause to constipation during pregnancy.

- Heartburn: Increased progesterone levels may relax the lower esophageal sphincter, resulting in acid reflux.

3. Postpartum Digestive Challenges:
- Hormonal Adjustments: After labor, hormonal variations may alter bowel patterns, and women may have constipation or irregularity.

- Pelvic Floor Issues: Changes in the pelvic floor after delivery might lead to digestive difficulties.

4. Menopause-Related Gut Problems:

- hormone Shifts: Menopausal hormone shifts might impact gut health, possibly leading to symptoms including bloating, constipation, or diarrhea.

- Osteoporosis and Gut Health: The reduction in estrogen during menopause may impair bone health, especially the bones of the digestive system.

5. IBS and Women:

- Prevalence: Irritable Bowel Syndrome (IBS) is more frequent in women, and hormonal variables may contribute to symptom changes over the menstrual cycle.

6. Gut Microbiota Changes:

- Hormonal Fluctuations: Hormonal changes throughout a woman's life, including puberty, pregnancy, and menopause, might impact the makeup of the gut microbiota.

7. Gynecological Surgeries and Digestive Health:

- Hysterectomy: Surgical removal of the uterus may occasionally lead to changes in bowel habits or digestive pain.

- Pelvic Surgeries: Procedures affecting the pelvic region might impair the function of surrounding digestive organs.

8. Stress and Digestive Issues in Women:

- Psychosocial Factors: Women may be more sensitive to stress-related digestive disorders, and stress management is critical for general gut health.

9. Eating Disorders and Women:

- Prevalence: Eating disorders, more frequent in women, may dramatically influence intestinal health and nutritional absorption.

10. Autoimmune Conditions:

- Gender Disparities: Some autoimmune disorders affecting the stomach, such as celiac disease, are more frequent in women.

CHAPTER 4

NOURISHING YOUR GUT

Nourishing your gut entails adopting dietary and lifestyle behaviors that promote the health and balance of your gut bacteria, leading to good digestion and general well-being. Here's a guide on feeding your gut:

1. Diverse and Fiber-Rich Diet:
- Colorful Vegetables and Fruits: Include a range of colorful vegetables and fruits in your diet to give a spectrum of nutrients and fiber.
- Whole Grains: Choose whole grains like quinoa, brown rice, and oats for added fiber.

2. Probiotic-Rich Foods:

- Yogurt and Fermented Foods: Incorporate yogurt, kefir, sauerkraut, kimchi, and other fermented foods high in probiotics to introduce good bacteria to your stomach.

3. Prebiotic-Rich Foods:

- Garlic, Onions, and Asparagus: Consume prebiotic-rich meals that support the existing beneficial bacteria in your stomach.

4. Healthy Fats:

- Avocados, Nuts, and Olive Oil: Include sources of healthy fats in your diet, such as avocados, almonds, seeds, and olive oil, which improve intestinal health.

5. Lean Proteins:

- Fish, Poultry, Legumes: Choose lean sources of protein, including fish, chicken, lentils, and plant-based proteins to maintain a balanced diet.

6. Hydration:

- Water Intake: Stay appropriately hydrated since water is vital for digestion, vitamin absorption, and maintaining the mucosal lining of the intestines.

7. Limit Processed Foods and Sugars:

- Whole, Unprocessed Foods: Minimize the consumption of processed foods and added sweets, since they may severely affect gut health.

8. Moderate Alcohol Consumption:
- Limit Intake: If you drink alcohol, do it in moderation, since excessive alcohol might upset the equilibrium of gut microorganisms.

9. Mindful Eating:
- Chew Thoroughly: Practice attentive eating by chewing your meal completely, assisting in improved digestion and nutritional absorption.

10. Regular Eating Schedule:

- Consistent Meal Times: Establish a regular eating schedule to assist the circadian rhythm and digestive functions.

12. Adequate Sleep:

- Prioritize Sleep: Ensure adequate and quality sleep, since sleep is vital for general health, including gut function.

13. Limit Antibiotic Use: - Judicious Use: Use antibiotics sparingly, since they may influence the balance of gut microorganisms. If prescribed, follow your healthcare provider's recommendations.

14. Consult with Healthcare Professionals: - Individualized Guidance: Seek counsel from

healthcare specialists, especially registered dietitians, for individualized recommendations based on your unique health requirements.

Dietary Guidelines for Gut Health

Dietary recommendations for gut health concentrate on promoting a varied and balanced gut flora, which is crucial for healthy digestion and general well-being. Incorporating a range of nutrient-rich meals and making conscious dietary choices may help to a healthy gut. Here are dietary tips for supporting intestinal health:

1. Diverse and Plant-Based Diet

2. Probiotic-Rich Foods:
- Yogurt, Kefir, and Fermented Foods: Include probiotic-rich foods in your diet, such as yogurt, kefir, sauerkraut, kimchi, and pickles, to introduce helpful bacteria to your stomach.

3. Prebiotic-Rich Foods

4. Healthy Fats

5. Lean Proteins: - Fish, Poultry, Legumes: Choose lean sources of protein, including

fish, chicken, lentils, and plant-based proteins to maintain a balanced diet.

6. Fiber Intake:

- Whole Plant Foods: Prioritize fiber-rich foods including fruits, vegetables, whole grains, and legumes. Fiber improves intestinal regularity and stimulates the development of healthy microorganisms.

7. Hydration

8. Limit Processed Foods and Sugars

9. Moderate Alcohol Consumption:

- Limit Intake: If you drink alcohol, do it in moderation, since excessive alcohol might upset the equilibrium of gut microorganisms.

10. Mindful Eating: - Chew Thoroughly: Practice attentive eating by chewing your meal completely, assisting in digestion and nutritional absorption.

11. Regular Eating Schedule

12. Proper Food Handling: - Food Safety Practices: Practice appropriate food handling and cleanliness to avoid infection and protect the health of your stomach.

13. Limit Antibiotic Use: - Judicious Use: Use antibiotics wisely, following your healthcare provider's directions, since they may influence the balance of gut flora.

14. Consider Individual Tolerances: - Identify Trigger Foods: Pay attention to how your body reacts to various meals and evaluate any intolerances or sensitivities you may have.

15. Seek Professional Guidance

Prebiotics and Probiotics

Prebiotics and probiotics serve vital roles in promoting healthy gut flora, regulating digestive health and general well-being. Understanding the difference between these two components is vital for integrating them into a balanced and gut-friendly diet.

Prebiotics:

Definition: Prebiotics are non-digestible fibers present in some meals that nourish and stimulate the development of beneficial bacteria in the stomach.

Sources: - Fruits: Bananas, apples, berries - Vegetables: Garlic, onions, asparagus -

Whole Grains: Oats, barley, quinoa - Legumes: Lentils, chickpeas

Benefits:

1. Feeding Beneficial Bacteria: Prebiotics serve as fuel for probiotics and other beneficial bacteria in the gut, encouraging their development and activity.

2. Enhanced Gut Barrier Function: They contribute to the formation and maintenance of a healthy gut lining, promoting barrier function and inhibiting the infiltration of hazardous chemicals.

Probiotics:

Definition: Probiotics are living microorganisms, typically bacteria and yeasts, that provide health advantages when taken in suitable concentrations.

Sources: - Yogurt: Contains strains like Lactobacillus and Bifidobacterium.
- Fermented Foods: Sauerkraut, kimchi, kefir, miso, and pickles.
- Supplements: Probiotic supplements with specialized strains for targeted health advantages.

Benefits:

1. Balancing Gut Microbiota: Probiotics bring helpful bacteria to the gut, helping maintain a healthy microbiota.

2. Digestive Health: They may improve symptoms of digestive disorders such as irritable bowel syndrome (IBS), diarrhea, and constipation.

3. Immune System Support: Probiotics may contribute to a stronger immune system by fostering a healthy gut environment.

4. Mental Health: Emerging research reveals a relationship between gut health and mental well-being, with probiotics possibly having a role in mental health support.

Considerations: - Strain Specificity: Different strains of probiotics may have varied effects, thus picking the proper strains for certain health objectives is vital.

- Storage: Probiotics are living organisms sensitive to conditions like heat and moisture, therefore correct storage is vital for ensuring their viability.

- Individual Responses: Responses to probiotics may vary, and their efficiency may rely on variables such as the individual's health situation and the exact strain eaten.

Synergy between Prebiotics and Probiotics:

- Symbiotic Relationship: Consuming both prebiotics and probiotics provides a synergistic impact, improving the survival and activity of beneficial bacteria in the stomach.

- Fermented Foods: Many fermented foods naturally include both prebiotics and probiotics, giving a holistic approach to gut health.

CHAPTER 5

LIFESTYLE AND GUT HEALTH

Lifestyle decisions have a crucial impact on defining the health of your gut. Adopting practices that encourage a healthy and robust gut flora benefits not just digestive health but also general well-being. Here are significant components of lifestyle that impact gut health:

1. Diet:

- Diversity of Foods: A diversified diet rich in fruits, vegetables, whole grains, lean meats, and healthy fats promotes a diverse gut flora.

- Prebiotics and Probiotics: Include prebiotic-rich foods (garlic, onions, bananas) and probiotic-containing foods (yogurt, kefir, fermented vegetables) to nourish and introduce good bacteria to the gut.

2. Stress Management:
- Mindfulness Practices: Engage in stress-reducing activities such as meditation, deep breathing, yoga, or mindfulness to lessen the effect of chronic stress on gut health.

- Balanced Lifestyle: Strive for a work-life balance and emphasize activities that offer relaxation and pleasure.

3. Physical exercise:

- Regular Exercise: Engage in regular physical exercise to increase gastrointestinal motility and general health. Exercise has been related to a more diversified gut microbiome.

   - Moderation is Key: Balance is key; excessive activity may have declining advantages on intestinal health.

 4. Adequate Sleep:

- Consistent Sleep Schedule: Maintain a regular sleep pattern to promote circadian rhythms, which regulate gastrointestinal activities.

   - Quality Sleep: Aim for quality sleep since inadequate or interrupted sleep may influence gut health and the microbiota.

5. Hydration:

- Adequate Water Intake: Stay well-hydrated since water is vital for digestion, vitamin absorption, and maintaining the mucosal lining of the intestines.

6. Avoiding Overuse of Antibiotics:

- Judicious Use: Use antibiotics only when required, since they may upset the equilibrium of gut microorganisms. Follow healthcare professionals' guidelines for effective antibiotic usage.

7. Avoiding Overconsumption of Alcohol:

- Moderation: Consume alcohol in moderation, since excessive intake might adversely influence the gut flora.

8. Avoiding Smoking:

- Quit Smoking: If you smoke, consider quitting, since smoking has been related to abnormalities in the gut flora.

9. Avoiding Environmental Toxins:

- Minimize Exposure: Reduce exposure to environmental toxins and chemicals that may influence gut health.

10. Gut-Brain Connection:

- Mind-Gut Axis: Recognize the bidirectional relationship between the stomach and brain.

Emotional well-being and mental health may impact gut function, and vice versa.

11. Regular Health Check-ups:
- Screening and Monitoring: Regular medical check-ups enable for monitoring of general health, including gut-related issues.

12. Probiotic and Lifestyle Synergy:
- Symbiotic Approach: Combine lifestyle decisions with the use of probiotics and prebiotics for a holistic approach to gut health.

The relationship between stress and gut health is a complicated dynamic that includes bidirectional communication between the brain and the stomach. Stress, whether acute or chronic, may have substantial impacts on the digestive system, altering both the gut microbiota and the general function of the gastrointestinal tract. Here's an investigation of the link between stress and intestinal health:

1. Gut-Brain Axis:

- Bi-Directional Communication: The gut and brain are linked via the gut-brain axis, a bidirectional communication system including the neurological, immunological, and endocrine systems.

- Effect of Emotions: Emotional states, especially stress, may affect gut function, and conversely, the gut can transmit signals that affect mood and emotions.

2. Effects of Stress on Digestive Processes:

- Altered Motility: Stress may lead to alterations in gut motility, perhaps causing diarrhea or constipation.

- Increased Permeability: Chronic stress may lead to increased intestinal permeability, frequently referred to as "leaky gut," enabling substances to flow through the intestinal barrier more readily.

3. Microbiota Influence:

- Microbiome Changes: Stress may change the makeup and diversity of the gut microbiota. Shifts in microbial balance may have ramifications for gut health.

- Impact on Beneficial Bacteria: Chronic stress may diminish the quantity of helpful bacteria while boosting the development of potentially dangerous microorganisms.

4. Stress-Induced Inflammation:

- Immune Response: Stress may stimulate the immune system, resulting to inflammation in the stomach. Chronic inflammation is connected with numerous digestive diseases.

5. Functional Gastrointestinal Disorders:

- Exacerbation of Symptoms: Stress is known to increase symptoms in patients with functional gastrointestinal diseases such as irritable bowel syndrome (IBS).

- Reciprocal connection: Individuals with persistent digestive difficulties may feel greater stress, producing a reciprocal connection.

6. Stress Management Strategies for Gut Health:

- Mindfulness Practices: Engage in mindfulness practices, meditation, and deep breathing to lessen the physiological effect of stress on the gut.

- Regular Physical Activity: Regular exercise is not only excellent for general well-being but also helps with stress reduction and increased gastrointestinal motility.

- Adequate Sleep: Prioritize adequate and quality sleep, since sleep loss may worsen stress and severely damage gut health.

7. Gut-Targeted Therapies:

- Probiotics: Certain probiotics may have potential advantages in controlling the gut-brain axis and lowering stress-induced alterations in the microbiota.

- Prebiotics: Prebiotic fibers may encourage the development of beneficial bacteria in the stomach, thereby decreasing the effect of stress.

8. Professional Support:

- Counseling and Therapy: Individuals suffering chronic stress influencing their gut health may benefit from counseling or therapy to address stresses and build coping techniques.

- Healthcare counsel: Consult healthcare specialists for individualized counsel, particularly if stress-related digestive difficulties continue.

Exercise and Gut Health

Exercise has a crucial role in supporting gut health, impacting numerous components of the digestive system and the gut flora. Regular physical exercise has been connected with a variety of advantages for the gastrointestinal system. Here's an investigation of the link between exercise and intestinal health:

1. Improved Gut Motility:

- Enhanced Peristalsis: Physical activity, especially aerobic exercise, increases peristalsis—the rhythmic contractions of the digestive tract which assists in the transportation of food through the intestines.

- Reduced Constipation: Regular exercise may treat constipation by generating regular bowel movements.

2. Impact on Gut Microbiota:

- Increased Microbial Diversity: Exercise has been related to an increase in the variety of the gut microbiota. A more diversified microbiome is connected with improved overall health.

- Promotion of Beneficial Bacteria: Some research shows that exercise may boost the development of beneficial bacteria in the gut.

3. Decreased Inflammation:

- Anti-Inflammatory Effects: Regular physical activity is linked with decreased inflammation throughout the body, including the stomach.

- Lower Risk of Inflammatory Bowel Diseases (IBD): Exercise has been associated with a decreased chance of acquiring inflammatory bowel disorders such as Crohn's disease and ulcerative colitis.

4. Stress Reduction:

- Stress Mitigation: Exercise is a potent stress reliever, and stress reduction is vital for maintaining gut health. High stress levels might significantly impair intestinal function.

- Positive Impact on Gut-Brain Axis: Exercise modulates the gut-brain axis, leading to a healthy communication system between the digestive system and the brain.

5. Weight Management:

- Keeping Healthy Weight: Regular physical activity improves weight management, and keeping a healthy weight is connected to improved gut health.

- Reduced Risk of Obesity-Related Gut Issues: Exercise may help minimize the risk of obesity-related digestive disorders such as non-alcoholic fatty liver disease (NAFLD).

6. Enhanced Insulin Sensitivity:

- Improved Blood Sugar Control: Exercise enhances insulin sensitivity, which may favorably influence blood sugar regulation and may lessen the chance of developing metabolic illnesses that affect the stomach.

7. Timing of Exercise and Digestion:

- Consideration of Meal Timing: Exercising at particular periods, such as post-meals, may alter digestion. Moderate-intensity exercise after a meal may assist in glucose metabolism.

8. Types of Exercise:

- Aerobic Exercise: Activities like jogging, cycling, or swimming have been related to good impacts on gut health.

- Resistance Training: Strength training activities may also help to better gut health.

9. Hydration and Exercise:

- Adequate Fluid Intake: Staying well-hydrated is vital during exercise to promote general health and digestive function.

10. Individualized Approach:

- Consideration of Individual Tolerance: The influence of exercise on gut health might differ across people, and it's crucial to adopt a regimen that meets personal preferences and tolerances.

CHAPTER 6

GUT HEALTH THROUGH THE LIFE STAGES

Gut health is a dynamic element of well-being that varies through several life phases, impacted by variables such as age, nutrition, lifestyle, and physiological changes. Understanding how gut health changes over time helps people to make educated decisions that promote optimum digestive function and overall well-being.

Here's an outline of gut health concerns during various life stages:

1. Infancy and Early Childhood:
- Establishing Microbiota: The early years are critical for building a diversified and robust gut flora. Factors like breastfeeding and exposure to a range of diets contribute to microbial diversity.
- Impact on Immune System: A healthy stomach in infancy fosters the development of the immune system, impacting long-term health.

2. Childhood and Adolescence:
- Dietary Habits: Introducing a balanced and diverse diet rich in fruits, vegetables, and

fiber throughout childhood improves continued gut health.

- Emphasis on Prebiotics: Including prebiotic-rich meals encourages the development of healthy bacteria in the gut.

- Influence of Lifestyle: Encouraging physical exercise and controlling stress favorably improves gut health throughout these early years.

3. Adulthood:

- Dietary Diversity: Maintaining a diversified and nutrient-rich diet helps gut microbiota stability.

- Preventive Measures: Healthy lifestyle choices, including regular exercise and stress management, become more crucial for preventing gut-related disorders.

- Probiotics and Prebiotics: Including probiotic and prebiotic foods may be helpful, particularly during times of stress or antibiotic usage.

4. Pregnancy:

- Microbiota Changes: Pregnancy may alter the gut microbiota, with possible modifications in microbial composition.

- Importance of Nutrition: Proper nutrition improves the health of both the mother and the growing baby, affecting gut health.

- Probiotic Supplementation: Some pregnant people may explore probiotic supplementation, with healthcare direction, to promote gut health.

5. Menopause and Beyond:

- Hormone Changes: Menopausal hormone changes might influence gut flora and may lead to digestive complaints.

- Bone Health and Gut Interaction: Supporting bone health via good diet and gastrointestinal health is critical during and after menopause.

- Probiotics and Hormonal Balance: Probiotics may have a role in promoting hormonal balance and gut health during menopausal transitions.

6. Older Adulthood:

- Nutrient Absorption: Aging may impair nutrient absorption in the gut, making dietary choices rich in vitamins and minerals vital.

- Fiber consumption: Adequate fiber consumption helps maintain bowel regularity, reducing constipation prevalent in elderly persons.

- Hydration: Ensuring appropriate hydration is crucial for digestive function, particularly since hydration demands may fluctuate with age.

7. Long-Term Strategies:

- Regular Health Check-ups: Routine health check-ups and screenings help detect and manage gut-related disorders early.

- Lifestyle Adaptations: Adjusting diet and lifestyle depending on changing health demands supports long-term gut health.

Pregnancy and Gut Health

Pregnancy brings about significant physiological changes, and these adaptations extend to the digestive system and intestinal health. The complicated interaction between hormonal variations, changes in food choices, and the changing gut flora during pregnancy demands particular study. Here's an investigation of the link between pregnancy and intestinal health:

1. Hormonal Impact on Digestion:
- Progesterone Levels: Elevated amounts of progesterone during pregnancy may lead to the relaxation of smooth muscles, particularly those in the digestive system. This may result in slower digestion and increased water absorption, perhaps causing constipation.

2. Gut Microbiota Changes:
- Shifts in Microbial Composition: Pregnancy is related to changes in the gut microbiota, mediated by hormonal swings and immune system responses.

- Microbial Diversity: Maintaining a varied gut microbiota during pregnancy is vital for general health, as microbial balance contributes to immune function and metabolic control.

3. Digestive Symptoms:
- Common Issues: Pregnant women commonly suffer digestive symptoms such as heartburn, indigestion, and constipation owing to hormonal and mechanical causes.

- Morning Sickness: Nausea and vomiting, generally known as morning sickness, may impact gut comfort and nutritional absorption.

4. Nutrient Absorption and Dietary Considerations:

- Increased Nutrient Demands: Pregnancy needs more nutrients, including folate, iron, and calcium. Ensuring appropriate nutrition absorption from the gut is critical for embryonic growth.

- Dietary Fiber: Adequate fiber consumption from fruits, vegetables, and whole grains helps avoid constipation and maintains gut health.

5. Probiotics and Gut Health During Pregnancy:

- Potential Benefits: Some studies show taking probiotics during pregnancy may favorably alter the gut microbiota, thereby lowering the risk of certain pregnancy-related problems.

- Consultation with Healthcare practitioners: Probiotic supplementation should be conducted with advice from healthcare practitioners to ensure safety and appropriateness.

6. Impact of Gestational Diabetes:

- Insulin Resistance and Gut Health: Gestational diabetes, defined by insulin resistance throughout pregnancy, may alter the gut flora. Managing blood sugar levels via food and exercise is vital.

7. Hydration and Gut Function:

- Fluid Requirements: Adequate hydration improves digestion, helps avoid constipation, and is needed for the increased blood volume associated with pregnancy.

8. Gut-Brain Axis and Emotional Well-being:
- Stress Management: Emotional well-being during pregnancy is connected to the gut-brain axis. Managing stress via relaxation methods and support networks favorably improves intestinal health.

9. Postpartum Gut Health:
- Recovery and Hormonal Changes: Postpartum, hormonal changes continue, influencing the digestive system.

Re-establishing a healthy gut flora with a balanced diet and possibly probiotic usage may promote healing.

10.   Consultation with Healthcare Professionals:

- Individualized Guidance: Pregnant adults should seek help from healthcare specialists, particularly obstetricians, and nutritionists, to address specific gut health problems and nutritional demands.

CHAPTER 7

RESTORING GUT HEALTH

Restoring gut health entails adopting targeted methods to foster a healthy and flourishing gut flora, support optimum digestive function, and boost overall well-being. Whether addressing problems like dysbiosis, inflammation, or other gut-related disorders, the following measures may aid in restoring and maintaining a healthy gut:

1. Dietary Interventions:

- Fiber-Rich meals: Incorporate a range of fiber-rich meals such as fruits, vegetables, and whole grains to feed good gut flora and encourage regular bowel movements.

- Prebiotic Foods: Include prebiotic-rich foods like garlic, onions, bananas, and asparagus to offer fuel for the development of helpful microorganisms.

- Probiotic Foods: Introduce probiotic-rich foods like yogurt, kefir, sauerkraut, kimchi, and pickles to raise the population of beneficial bacteria.

2. Elimination and Reintroduction:
- Identify Trigger Meals: Determine whether particular meals contribute to digestive pain and try temporarily removing possible triggers.

- Gradual Reintroduction: Reintroduce removed foods gradually to discover unique triggers and learn individual tolerances.

3. Probiotic Supplements:

- Consultation with Healthcare practitioners: Consider probiotic supplements under the supervision of healthcare practitioners, particularly if specific strains are indicated for targeted health advantages.

- Quality and Strain Selection: Choose high-quality probiotic supplements with strains that correspond with particular health objectives.

4. Prebiotic Supplements:

- Supplement Wisely: Consider prebiotic supplements to boost the development of healthy microorganisms.

  - Start Slowly: Begin with a modest dosage and gradually increase to reduce any gastric discomfort.

5. Anti-Inflammatory Diet:

- Omega-3 Fatty Acids: Include foods rich in omega-3 fatty acids, such as fatty fish and flaxseeds, to help decrease inflammation.

  - Colorful Antioxidant-Rich Foods: Consume a range of colorful fruits and vegetables for their antioxidant effects.

6. Stress Management:

- Mindfulness Practices: Engage in stress-reducing activities like meditation, deep breathing, or yoga to favorably influence the gut-brain axis.

- Regular Physical Activity: Incorporate regular exercise, which has been linked to better gut health and lower stress.

7. Hydration:

- Adequate Water Intake: Stay well-hydrated to assist digestion, nutritional absorption, and the health of the mucosal lining of the intestines.

8. Antibiotic Use:

- Probiotic Supplementation During Antibiotics: If given antibiotics, consider taking probiotic supplements to help reduce disturbances to the gut flora.

- Follow Healthcare Provider's Recommendations: Adhere to healthcare professionals' directions about antibiotic usage.

9. Individualized Approach:

- Consideration of Personal Factors: Tailor therapies depending on individual health status, preferences, and unique gut health issues.

- Professional Guidance: Consult with healthcare specialists, particularly qualified dietitians or gastroenterologists, for individualized recommendations.

10. Regular Monitoring:

- Listen to Body Signals: Pay attention to how the body reacts to food and lifestyle changes.

- Adjust as Needed: Make modifications depending on continuing observations and input from the body.

11. Seeking Professional Support:

- Gastroenterologist or Registered Dietitian

Gut Healing Protocols

Gut healing protocols are comprehensive procedures aimed at treating and relieving numerous gut-related disorders, encouraging the restoration of healthy gut flora, and supporting normal digestive function. These programs frequently comprise a mix of dietary, behavioral, and supplemental treatments. Here's an outline of essential components often found in gut healing protocols:

1. Elimination Diet:

- Identification of Trigger Foods: Begin with an elimination phase to identify and eliminate possible trigger foods that may contribute to digestive troubles.

- Common Elimination Targets: Dairy, gluten, some cereals, and highly processed meals are commonly evaluated during this time.

2. Anti-Inflammatory Diet:

- Emphasis on Whole Foods: Focus on a diet rich in whole, nutrient-dense foods such as fruits, vegetables, lean proteins, and healthy fats.

- Omega-3 Fatty Acids: Incorporate foods rich in omega-3 fatty acids, such as fatty fish and flaxseeds, to decrease inflammation.

3. Bone Broth:

- Collagen and Amino Acids: Bone broth is rich in collagen and amino acids, which may help gut lining integrity and healing.

4. Probiotics:

- Multi-Strain Supplements: Introduce high-quality probiotic supplements with a range of strains to stimulate the development of beneficial bacteria.

- Probiotic-Rich Foods: Incorporate fermented foods like yogurt, kefir, sauerkraut, and kimchi for extra probiotic assistance.

5. Prebiotics:

- Prebiotic-Rich Foods: Include foods high in prebiotic fibers, such as garlic, onions, bananas, and asparagus, to support good gut flora.

6. Digestive Enzymes:

- Supplementation: Consider digestive enzyme supplements to assist in the breakdown and absorption of nutrients, particularly if there are digestion issues.

7. L-Glutamine Supplementation:

- Support for Gut Lining: L-Glutamine, an amino acid, is considered to enhance the integrity of the gut lining and may help in its repair.

8. Aloe Vera:

- Anti-Inflammatory Properties: Aloe vera is occasionally utilized for its anti-inflammatory qualities and possible help for gut repair.

9. Slippery Elm:

- Mucilage Content: Slippery elm, with its mucilage content, may help calm and protect the digestive system.

10. Gut-Supportive Herbs:

- Chamomile, Marshmallow Root: Herbs like chamomile and marshmallow root are sometimes used for their possible calming effects on the digestive tract.

11. Gradual Reintroduction:

healthcare specialists. Here's an overview of vitamins usually related to intestinal health:

1. Probiotics:

- Considerations: Different strains provide varying health advantages, thus talking with healthcare specialists helps establish the most effective probiotic for individual requirements.

2. Prebiotics:

- Considerations: While prebiotics are naturally available in meals, supplements may be explored under expert direction to guarantee optimal consumption.

3. Digestive Enzymes: - Definition: Digestive enzymes help in the breakdown of macronutrients (proteins, lipids, carbs) into smaller, absorbable components.

- Function: Supplements may improve digestion, especially in persons with enzyme deficits or digestive problems.

- Sources: Available in supplement form, with varied formulas addressing certain digestion requirements.

4. L-Glutamine: - Function: L-Glutamine is an amino acid thought to enhance the integrity and repair of the gut lining.

- Sources: Available as a supplement or naturally found in some foods such as cattle, poultry, fish, dairy, and certain plant-based sources.

- Considerations: Consultation with healthcare specialists is required, since excessive ingestion may have detrimental consequences.

5. Aloe Vera:

- Sources: Available as a supplement or in gel form from the inner leaf of the aloe vera plant.

- Considerations: Moderation is necessary, and expert advice is advised.

6. Fish Oil (Omega-3 Fatty Acids):

- Considerations: Dosage and quality of supplements should be addressed with healthcare practitioners.

7. Fiber Supplements: - Function: Fiber maintains digestive regularity and feeds good gut flora.

- Sources: Fiber supplements like psyllium husk or methylcellulose.

- Considerations: Adequate water consumption is necessary while eating fiber supplements to avoid constipation.

8. Collagen: - Function: Collagen supplements may enhance the integrity of the gut lining and connective tissues.

- Sources: Collagen peptides obtained from animal or fish sources.

- Considerations: Consultation with healthcare experts is encouraged, particularly for people with allergies or sensitivities.

9. Vitamin D: - Function: Adequate vitamin D levels are connected with a healthy gut microbiome.

- Sources: Sunlight exposure, food sources, and supplementation.

- Considerations: Vitamin D supplementation should be individualized depending on individual requirements and levels.

10. Magnesium: - Function: Magnesium aids muscular relaxation, especially the muscles of the digestive tract.

- Sources: Dietary sources and supplements.

- Considerations: Excessive ingestion may cause diarrhea; dose should be controlled.

11. Zinc: - Function: Zinc has a role in maintaining the intestinal barrier and immunological function.

- Sources: Dietary sources and supplements. - Considerations: Consultation with healthcare specialists is crucial since excessive zinc consumption might have detrimental consequences.

12. Consultation with Healthcare Providers:

- Individualized Approach: The requirement and suitability of supplements vary depending on individual health state.

- Monitoring and modifications: Regular interaction with healthcare specialists enables correct monitoring and modifications to supplement regimens.

Chapter 8

RECIPES FOR GUT HEALTH

Promoting intestinal health with a well-balanced and healthy diet is crucial. Here are a few dishes that use foods recognized for their gut-friendly properties:

1. **Probiotic-Rich Smoothie Bowl**:
Ingredients:
   - 1 cup yogurt (Greek)
 - 1 cup mixed berries (blueberries, strawberries)
- 1 banana
   - 1 tablespoon chia seeds
   - 1 tablespoon honey
   - Granola for topping
Instructions:
   1. Blend yogurt, mixed berries, banana, chia seeds, and honey until smooth.
   2. Pour into a bowl and top with granola for additional fiber.

2. **Quinoa and Vegetable Stir-Fry**:
Ingredients:
 - 1 cup cooked quinoa
 - Mixed veggies (bell peppers, broccoli, carrots)
- 1 tablespoon olive oil
    - 2 cloves garlic (minced)
    - 1 teaspoon ginger (grated)
    - Soy sauce to taste
 Instructions:
    1. garlic and ginger in olive oil.
    2. Add mixed veggies and stir-fry until tender.
    3. Mix in cooked quinoa and soy sauce. Serve warm.

3. **Salmon and Avocado Salad**:
 Ingredients:
 - Grilled salmon fillet
- Mixed greens (spinach, arugula)
- Cherry tomatoes, halved
    - Avocado, sliced
    - Lemon vinaigrette dressing
Instructions:
    1. Grill fish until cooked.

2. Assemble a salad with mixed greens, cherry tomatoes, avocado, and grilled salmon.

3. Drizzle with lemon vinaigrette dressing.

4. **Chia Seed Pudding**:

Ingredients:

  - 3 tablespoons chia seeds
- 1 cup almond milk
- 1 teaspoon honey
- Fresh fruit for topping

Instructions:

1. Mix chia seeds with almond milk. Let it rest in the refrigerator for a few hours or overnight.

2. Stir in honey and top with fresh fruit before serving.

5. **Roasted Sweet Potato and Lentil Soup**:

Ingredients:

  - 2 sweet potatoes (peeled and chopped)
  - 1 cup red lentils
  - 1 onion (chopped)
  - 2 cloves garlic (minced)
  - 1 teaspoon turmeric

- 1 teaspoon cumin
    - 4 cups veggie broth
Instructions:
    1. Roast sweet potatoes till tender.
    2. Sauté onions and garlic until softened.
    3. Add roasted sweet potatoes, red lentils, turmeric, cumin, and vegetable broth.
    4. Simmer until the lentils are done. Blend until smooth.

6. **Fermented Vegetable Medley**:
Ingredients:
    - Assorted veggies (carrots, cucumbers, radishes)
    - 1 tablespoon sea salt
    - Water
Instructions:
    1. Slice veggies and place them into a jar.
    2. Dissolve sea salt in water and sprinkle over the veggies.
    3. Close the jar and let it ferment at room temperature for a few days.

7. Turmeric Ginger Tea:

Ingredients:
- 1 teaspoon turmeric (freshly grated or powder)
- 1 teaspoon ginger (freshly grated)
- 1 tablespoon honey
- 1 lemon (juiced)
- 2 cups hot water

Instructions:

1. Mix turmeric, ginger, honey, and lemon juice in boiling water.

2. Stir thoroughly and enjoy this anti-inflammatory tea.

Tips: - Include Fiber: Opt for whole grains, fruits, and vegetables rich in soluble and insoluble fiber. - Limit Processed Foods: Minimize consumption of processed and sugary foods that might adversely affect gut health.

- Stay Hydrated: Water is necessary for digestion and general gut health.

Gut-Friendly Meal Plan

Day 1:

Breakfast: Probiotic Smoothie Bowl

- 1 cup yogurt (Greek or plant-based)

- 1/2 cup mixed berries (blueberries, raspberries)

- 1 banana

- 1 tablespoon chia seeds

- Topped with granola and a honey drizzle

Lunch: Quinoa and Vegetable Stir-Fry

- 1 cup cooked quinoa - Mixed veggies (bell peppers, broccoli, carrots)

- 1 tablespoon olive oil - 2 cloves garlic
(minced)
- Soy sauce to taste

Snack: Fresh Fruit Salad - Variety of
seasonal fruits (watermelon, pineapple, kiwi)
- Optional: sprinkle with chia seeds

Dinner: Baked Salmon with Roasted Sweet
Potatoes
- Grilled salmon fillet - Roasted sweet potato
cubes with olive oil and rosemary - Mixed
greens salad with a lemon vinaigrette
dressing

Day 2:

Breakfast: Chia Seed Pudding Parfait - 3 tablespoons chia seeds combined with almond milk - Layered with yogurt and topped with fresh berries

Lunch: Lentil and Vegetable Soup - Red lentils, carrots, celery, onion, garlic, turmeric, cumin, vegetable broth - Serve with a piece of whole-grain bread

Snack: Fermented Vegetable Medley - Assorted fermented veggies (carrots, cucumbers, radishes)

Dinner: Grilled Chicken Salad - Grilled chicken breast - Mixed greens, cherry tomatoes, cucumber, and avocado

- Olive oil and balsamic vinegar dressing

Day 3:

Breakfast: Avocado Toast with Poached Eggs
- Whole-grain toast with mashed avocado
- Poached eggs on top - Sprinkle with salt, pepper, and a splash of paprika

Lunch: Quinoa Salad with Roasted Vegetables - Quinoa, roasted zucchini, cherry tomatoes, red onion - Feta cheese and a sprinkle of balsamic glaze

Snack: Greek Yogurt Parfait - Greek yogurt with honey and a handful of nuts

Dinner: Turkey and Vegetable Stir-Fry

- Ground turkey, mixed veggies, ginger, garlic

- Soy sauce and sesame oil for taste

- Served over brown rice

 Tips for a Gut-Friendly Diet:

Include Probiotics: Incorporate probiotic-rich foods including yogurt, kefir, sauerkraut, and kimchi.

- Fiber-Rich Foods: Choose whole grains, fruits, and vegetables to enhance intestinal health.

- Hydrate: Drink lots of water throughout the day to promote digestion.

- Limit Processed Foods: Minimize processed and sugary foods that may affect intestinal equilibrium.

- Balanced Meals: Aim for balanced meals with a combination of lean proteins, healthy fats, and a range of colorful veggies.

Remember to listen to your body and alter portion amounts depending on individual requirements. If you have special dietary problems or health issues, speak with a healthcare expert or a qualified dietitian for tailored guidance.

Cooking for Optimal Digestive Health

Cooking for optimum digestive health entails choosing products and preparing meals that encourage a healthy and well-functioning digestive tract. Here are some tips and ideas to boost intestinal health via cooking:

1. Choose Gut-Friendly Ingredients: - Whole Grains: Opt for whole grains like quinoa, brown rice, and oats for their fiber content that encourages regular bowel movements.

- Lean Proteins: Include lean protein sources such as chicken, fish, tofu, and lentils to offer needed amino acids without extra saturated fat.

2. Incorporate Fiber-Rich Foods: - Vegetables: Include a range of colorful vegetables in your meals. Broccoli, carrots, leafy greens, and bell peppers are wonderful alternatives.

- Fruits: Incorporate fresh fruits like berries, apples, and pears for extra fiber and natural sweetness.

3. Include Probiotic-Rich Foods: - Yogurt and Fermented Foods: Incorporate yogurt with live cultures, kefir, sauerkraut, and kimchi to incorporate important probiotics into your diet.

4. Healthy Fats: - Avocado: Avocado is rich in monounsaturated fats and fiber, promoting overall digestive health.

- Olive Oil: Use extra virgin olive oil for cooking and topping salads. It includes anti-inflammatory effects.

5. Cooking Techniques: - Steaming: Steaming veggies keeps their nutrients and makes them simpler to digest.

- Grilling and Baking: Choose grilling or baking techniques over frying to decrease extra oil and fat levels.

6. Herbs and Spices: - Ginger: Known for its anti-inflammatory effects, ginger may be used in soups, stir-fries, or teas.

- Turmeric: Contains curcumin, which has anti-inflammatory and antioxidant benefits. Use in curries, soups, or golden milk.

7. Hydration: - Water-Rich Foods: Include foods with high water content, such as cucumber and watermelon, to contribute to general hydration.

- Herbal Teas: Chamomile, peppermint, and ginger drinks might ease the digestive system.

8. Limit Processed Foods: - Reduce Added Sugars: Minimize the consumption of processed meals with added sugars, since they may upset the equilibrium of gut flora.

9. Meal Timing: - Regular Meals: Stick to regular meal times to assist manage digestion. Avoid heavy meals close before sleep.

10. Individual Considerations: - Food Sensitivities: Identify and manage any food sensitivities or intolerances that may contribute to digestive pain.

- Consultation with Professionals: If digestive troubles continue, speak with a healthcare practitioner or a certified dietitian for tailored counsel.

11. Digestive-Friendly Recipes: - Quinoa and Vegetable Stir-Fry: Packed with fiber and

veggies, this meal is light and simple to digest.

- Salmon with Lemon and Dill: Fatty fish like salmon contains omega-3 fatty acids and is pleasant on the stomach.

- Greek Yogurt Parfait with Berries and Almonds: A probiotic-rich dessert or snack.

Cooking for optimum digestive health is a comprehensive approach that incorporates nutritional quality, cooking techniques, and individual tastes. Tailoring your meals to promote digestion may add to overall well-being and comfort.

CONCLUSION

In conclusion, this trip through "Restoring Gut Health for Women" has been an investigation of the delicate link between gut health and general well-being. We've dug into the significance of a balanced diet, conscious living choices, and proactive ways to build a flourishing gut ecosystem.

As you negotiate the challenges of maintaining good gut health, remember that it's a dynamic and unique process. The ideas discussed in this book are not simply instructions but tools for you to adjust to your requirements. Your gut health is a sign of your dedication to self-care and a tribute to the resiliency of your body.

By emphasizing the well-being of your digestive system, you're investing in prolonged energy and general health. Whether you are attempting to heal, maintain, or avoid gut disorders, the answer lies in the consistency of your decisions and the awareness with which you approach your lifestyle.

As you continue your path, keep aware, stay proactive, and most importantly, stay receptive to the messages your body offers. Your digestive health is a continuous relationship between you and your body one that contains the potential to favorably affect every area of your life.

May your road to gut health be one of empowerment, exploration, and continued energy. Here's to a future where your gut flourishes, and so do you.

Achieving and Sustaining Gut Health

Achieving and maintaining gut health is a dynamic and gratifying process that involves dedication, awareness, and tailored tactics. As we complete our investigation of "Restoring Gut Health for Women," let's focus on the concrete activities and mentality required to obtain and sustain maximum digestive well-being.

Consistency is Key: The decisions you make every day greatly affect your gut health. Whether it's the meals you eat, the stress management tactics you utilize, or the lifestyle habits you embrace, consistency is crucial. Small, sustained adjustments over time may lead to big gains in your gut health.

Listen to Your Body: Your body communicates its wants, and listening to these messages is vital. Pay attention to how various meals make you feel, recognize stress triggers, and be mindful of the influence of your lifestyle on your digestive well-being. This self-awareness helps you to make educated decisions that match your body's necessities.

Evolve Your Approach: Recognize that establishing and keeping gut health is not a one-size-fits-all task. Your body develops, and so should your approach to gut health. Periodically examine your food and lifestyle habits, consider any changes in your living circumstances, and alter your methods appropriately.

Educate Yourself Continuously: Gut health is an area of continuing study, and new ideas arise constantly. Stay updated on the newest happenings, but approach information cautiously. Use the information to influence your choices, but allow your body's reactions to be the final guidance.

Celebrate Progress, Not Perfection: Achieving optimum gut health is not about perfection; it's about progress. Celebrate the wonderful changes you make, no matter how tiny. Acknowledge that setbacks may occur, and regard them as chances to learn and alter your approach.

Holistic Well-Being Matters: Gut health is directly tied to your overall well-being. Practices like mindfulness, adequate sleep, and positive relationships contribute not only to a healthy gut but also to a fulfilling life.

Empower Yourself: You are the main champion for your health. Work together with healthcare providers, seek direction, and actively engage in choices surrounding your well-being. Empower yourself with information, follow your intuition, and take ownership of your path toward prolonged gut health.

Empowering Women Through Gut Health

Empowering women via gut health is more than simply encouraging digestive wellness; it's about understanding the significant influence that a healthy gut can have on overall empowerment, confidence, and energy. As we complete our investigation of "Restoring Gut Health for Women," let's look into the transforming impact of gut health in empowering women.

Physical Empowerment: A well-nourished and balanced stomach immediately impacts physical vigor. By adopting a nutrient-rich diet and gut-friendly activities, women may boost their physical well-being, fostering strength, resilience, and a feeling of physical empowerment that positively impacts everyday life.

Mental and Emotional Resilience: The gut-brain link is a significant conduit that impacts mental and emotional well-being. Nurturing a healthy gut flora leads to emotional resilience, stress management, and mental clarity. Empowered women make conscious decisions that promote not just their physical health but also their mental and emotional strength.

Confidence in Food decisions: Understanding the influence of food on gut health helps women to make educated and confident decisions regarding their diet. This information reduces guessing, allowing consumers to pick meals that match their body's demands and contribute to continuous well-being.

Balancing Hormones and Mood: Hormonal balance is tightly related to gut health, altering mood, energy levels, and general vitality. Women empowered via gut health may employ practices that promote hormonal balance, leading to more energy, better mood, and a feeling of control over their emotional well-being.

Self-Advocacy in Healthcare: A woman who knows her gut health can be a proactive champion for her overall health. By actively engaging in healthcare choices, seeking assistance, and prioritizing preventative care, she takes responsibility for her well-being and becomes a powerful force in her health journey.

Community and Support Networks: Empowerment is magnified in a supportive community. Women sharing their gut health experiences, thoughts, and tactics build a network of mutual support and encouragement. This feeling of community creates empowerment, emphasizing the belief that every woman's health journey is worthy and worthwhile.

Lifestyle as a Tool for Empowerment: Gut health becomes a tool for empowerment when it fits with a woman's lifestyle objectives. Whether pursuing a profession, managing a family, or participating in personal hobbies, a healthy gut offers the basis for continuous energy, attention, and endurance, helping women in reaching their ambitions.

Holistic wellbeing: An empowered woman realizes that well-being goes beyond physical health. By adopting a holistic approach that spans physical, mental, and emotional well-being, she cultivates a lifestyle that not only promotes a healthy gut but also adds to an overall feeling of empowerment and satisfaction.